IMPROVING THE DOCTOR - PATIENT RELATIONSHIP

A GUIDE FOR PHYSICIANS AND MEDICAL STUDENTS

by

Carmen M. Richards, M.D.
Fernando M. Siles, M. D.

Illustrated by: William Freeman, Ph.D.
Foreward by: Gerald G. Jampolsky, M.D.

IMPROVING THE DOCTOR - PATIENT RELATIONSHIP

A GUIDE FOR PHYSICIANS AND MEDICAL STUDENTS

by
Carmen M. Richards, M.D.
Fernando M. Siles, M. D.

Cover Design by: Rob D. Wipprecht
Illustrated by: William Freeman, Ph.D.

Published by

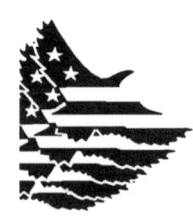

Blue Bird Publishing
1739 E. Broadway #306
Tempe AZ 85282
(602) 968-4088 (602) 831-6063

© 1995 by Carmen M. Richards and Fernando M. Siles
All rights reserved.

ISBN 0-933025-41-6 $11.95

Contents

Acknowledgments	4
Authors' Note	5
Foreward by Gerald Jampolsky, M.D.	6
Introduction	9
Factors That Affect the Doctor-Patient Relationship	11
Modern Medical Technology	12
The Fast Pace of Medical Practice	13
The Physician's Communication Skills	16
The Physician's Own Sense of Omnipotence	18
The Personality of the Physician	19
The Threat of Malpractice Suits	31
Work Overload and Stress	32
The Physician's Unconscious Feelings	35
The Physician's Own Health Problems	41
The Emergency Room Physician	52
The Doctor's Professional and Domestic Life	54
Ethical Boundaries	59
Conclusions	65
Recommendations	73
Closing Thoughts	77
Appendix I: Improve Your Practice with Better Communications by Dr. Neil Baum	83

ACKNOWLEDGMENTS

We want to express our gratitude to *Bill Freeman* for his creative illustrations, a generous contribution to this book.

We are also indebted to *John Richards* for the long hours that he spent reviewing and editing this work.

In addition, this book would not have been possible without *Laly Siles*, who worked dilligently in retyping, organizing and transferring the manuscript from one computer system to another.

AUTHORS' NOTE

This book is the result of many hours of reflective work analyzing the weakness of the medical profession in our days. The ideas expressed herein are a product of inspiration guided by the introspective view of ourselves.

We hope that the message of "rehumanizing" our profession will be well-received by fellow physicians and that those who read this work will become better communicators with themselves and with their patients as well.

FOREWARD

Gerald Jampolsky, M.D.
Author: Love is Letting Go of Fear

In this book the authors have captured essential aspects explaining the fundamentals underlying the communications between the doctor and his patient. The main idea expressed in this practical and insightful manual is that the healing process must first take place in the physician's consciousness. The power of love in the doctor's life is well presented by Dr. Richards and Dr. Siles. There is a strong conviction in their minds that ultimately all the endeavors in the medical profession, and the world as well, must be permeated by the sense of LOVE.

I firmly believe that the reader will benefit from the teachings of this book. Anyone who truly understands its empathic message will not be the same at the end of its reading.

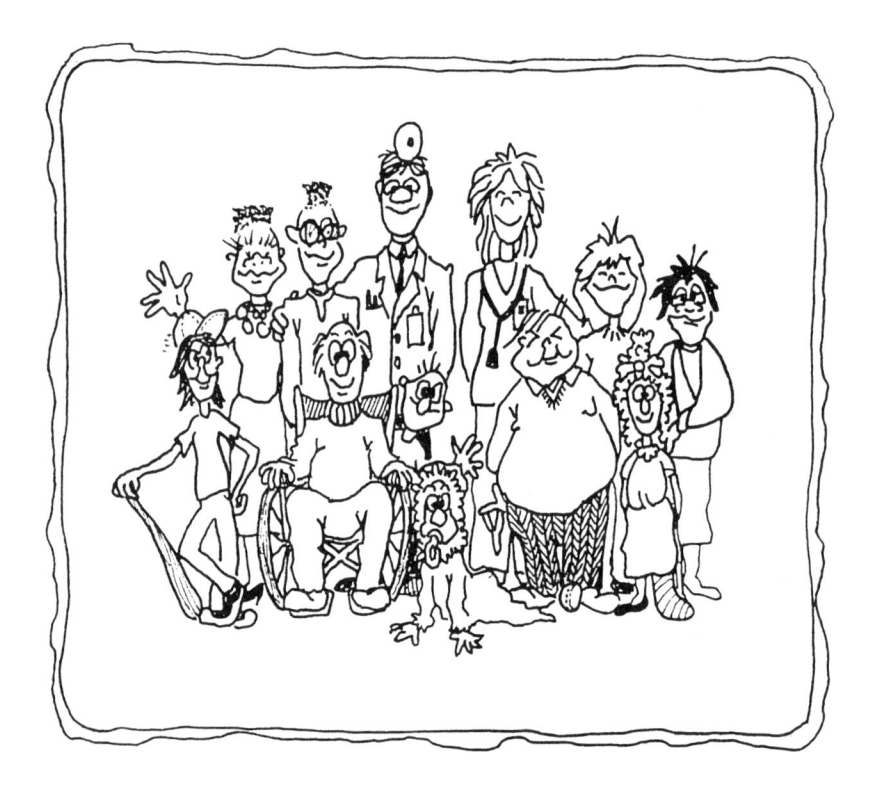

8   *Doctor-Patient Relationship*

INTRODUCTION

This book is intended for medical students, physicians and people in general. Its purpose is to provide them with information to help understand and improve the doctor-patient relationship.

This subject is of great importance for professionals in the medical field. Today, when modern society seems lost in its existential difficulties, doctors constantly need to be reminded about their important role as caregivers of human life and health. We, as physicians, are the professionals from whom patients expect to obtain reassurance, compassion, hope and love before they receive the highly advanced technical care which modern medicine provides.

Everyone who faces a health problem experiences a certain degree of insecurity about the nature and outcome of the illness. These feelings mobilize anxiety, depression and a sense of inadequacy that are expressed by the patient's attitude and behavior. Therefore, regardless of the nature of the illness and even if the disease is incurable or a product of somatization, the patient is in need of recciving supportive care from his physician.

Some of the medical schools now include in their curriculum courses on communication skills. This is much needed since the tendency of medical students is to apply themselves to the technical aspects of medicine and forget about its human side. Additionally, due to the academic demands of modern medical education, students often miss the opportunity to develop their social skills.

We are also observing a definite change in the life style of physicians. Currently there are more sub-specialties, less family doctors and almost no house calls. This too has had its negative impact on the human side of medicine.

In the next pages you will learn about the key factors which affect the doctor-patient relationship and gain insight into how physicians can continue to improve their ability to relate to patients.

FACTORS THAT AFFECT THE DOCTOR-PATIENT RELATIONSHIP

There are numerous factors that affect the doctor-patient relationship.

Among these are:

- Modern medical technology
- The fast pace of medical practice
- The physician's communication skills
- The physician's own sense of omnipotence
- The personality of the physician
- The threat of malpractice suits
- Work overload and stress
- The physician's unconscious feelings
- The physician's own health problems

Each of these deserves to be examined and understood.

MODERN MEDICAL TECHNOLOGY

In the last few decades, medical technology has achieved remarkable advances in the development of diagnostic tools as well as treatment modalities. We have become much more effective in detecting diseases and better able to alleviate symptoms or even heal nosological conditions. But it seems that all this improvement is basically focused on protecting the patient's body. We are in danger of denying the need, first of all, to take the patient's feelings into consideration.

Physicians tend to strive to render "the best of their services." By doing so, they may concentrate excessively on the mechanical and technical aspects of medical care. It is important to remember that patients respond better to the treatment provided when they perceive their physician has a sincere desire to understand their complaints. We must remind ourselves that we are treating patients and not illnesses.

THE FAST PACE OF MEDICAL PRACTICE

In most physician's offices the patient's first encounter is with the receptionist who gives a questionnaire to be filled out. They next meet with the nurse or medical technician in charge of administering various tests. Then comes what is all too often a brief contact with the doctor. During this time the physician must formulate his conclusions, order specialized tests, discuss prospective surgical interventions, prescribe medications and make further inquiry from the patient. In general, everything is done as fast as possible with little chance for an open discussion of the questions that the patient may have in mind.

When patients have an appointment with a physician, they expect to obtain answers to questions related to their health problems. They intend to communicate effectively with the doctor. They need to elucidate their most profound doubts. They want to have the opportunity to verbalize their fears and doubts involving the symptoms that brought them to the office. Sometimes, with concerned listening and empathic explanation by the doctor, the simple verbalization by the patient is sufficient to resolve ailments that are apparently serious from the patient's point of

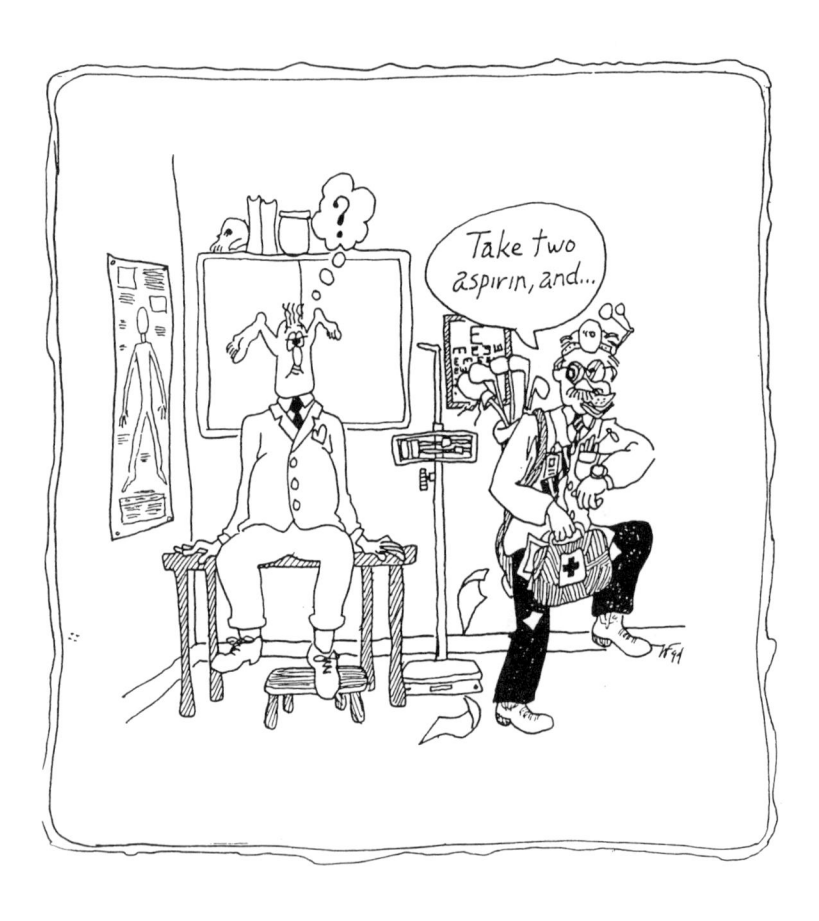

Doctor-Patient Relationship

view. If the patient is not encouraged to verbalize, he or she may end up leaving the physician's office with a distorted interpretation of what was verbalized or not verbalized by the doctor.

THE PHYSICIAN'S COMMUNICATION SKILLS

Communication among people is often impaired. The doctor-patient relationship involves peculiar aspects that make communication even more difficult. The patient tends to see the physician as a charismatic figure from whom he expects "magic solutions" or at least a message of hope that "everything will be solved or remedied." Because of this it is of great importance to emphasize the healing qualities of the spoken language.

Physicians need to encourage their patients to verbalize their thoughts and feelings frankly, without being inhibited, intimidated or frightened by the doctor's "powerful" position. The doctor needs to confirm that the patient understands the explanations he is given about his treatment. This is important because the perception of the patient's objective reality may be influenced by fears, beliefs, needs and wishes. The dialogue between physicians and patients will be more effective when it is based on a clear comprehension of the patient's subjective as well as objective world. When this is done, the instructions given to the patient for the therapeutic plan will be free of ambiguities and uncertainties.

In reality patients do not care as much about the physician "being a genius," when it comes to getting rid of their problems. They are mainly concerned about having a well balanced, caring, loving and competent doctor who will heal them, if possible, and mitigate their suffering whenever needed.

It is not always possible to cure a disease, but it is often feasible to alleviate the symptoms, sometimes just with the proper attention by the doctor. Consolation with a palliative gesture can best be accomplished when the physician is able to express love and compassion. This is not always easy. Physicians who were raised in homes where there was lack of expression of love and warm feelings have particular difficulties in communicating with their patients.

Some physicians do not even have basic communication skills, such as making direct eye contact when conversing with clients. They may feel threatened by closeness and often choose to talk to their patients from behind the desk. Doctors who feel vulnerable in this area may unconsciously decide to keep a fast pace during consultation in order to protect themselves from being exposed to their patients.

THE PHYSICIAN'S OWN SENSE OF OMNIPOTENCE

It is a well known fact that many physicians develop a sense of omnipotence. They realize that they are entitled to make very important decisions that have a great impact on their patient's lives, at times even involving life or death. This can cause doctors to protect themselves behind a mask of arrogance and false superiority and thus widen the gap between them and the patients.

Once doctors are able to work on their emotional frailties as human beings, they can improve their ability to communicate effectively with their patients. They can then realize that the most important figure in this dual relationship is the patient and not themselves. To help the patient, physicians need to deal with the narcissistic aspects of their own personalities. They must learn how to exercise the quality of being humble in order to express compassion, love and genuine concern for the patient's well-being.

When doctors are able to deal with their own internal limitations and difficulties, they will not be preoccupied with showing power and superiority towards the patient. By acting with modesty and by not trying to impress the patient with their expertise they will be better able to help.

THE PERSONALITY OF THE PHYSICIAN

Patients are most likely to benefit from the action of medications or to improve the quality of their behavior when they perceive the physician has a sincere desire to understand their problems. They can tell when the doctor is really concern with healing them. As a consequence they are more cooperative with medical workers who have a friendly and committed attitude towards them. On the contrary, opposite conduct (even unconsciously) in regards to the treatment can be expressed when the patient perceives the physician as distant or lacking humanitarian love.

Patients have the tendency to idealize the physician and tolerate poorly finding out that the doctor, as a human being, can have frailties. At the same time, when the doctor has certain personality traits, the patient can become easily aware of them. These negative personal characteristics play a key role in the quality of the doctor-patient relationship. Here are examples of the most common personality traits among physicians.

Obsessive-Compulsive Personality Traits

The majority of physicians fit this profile. Having obsessive-compulsive features helps them to succeed in medical school. Indeed, most patients appreciate these traits, which can be best noted when they make comments such as "the doctor was very thorough during the physical examination." The pitfall is that, when the physician is too compulsive, he or she may pay excessive attention to details and technical issues rather than to the patient. It is not unusual to find doctors who work long hours, mainly due to their obsessive character, as they take extra time in accomplishing each task of their daily work.

Physicians with obsessive-compulsive personality traits are in danger of focusing mostly on doing well and therefore, forgetting the fact that the patient is the central figure.

Narcissistic Personality Traits

Doctors with these traits have a tendency to overconcentrate on their own professional development and are not "patient oriented." When having contact with clients, family members and other professionals, they strive to be recognized as being brilliant and outstanding. They often have an excessive display of medical diplomas in their offices and tend to use unnecessary technical language when explaining procedures or side effects of prescribed medication.

Doctor-Patient Relationship

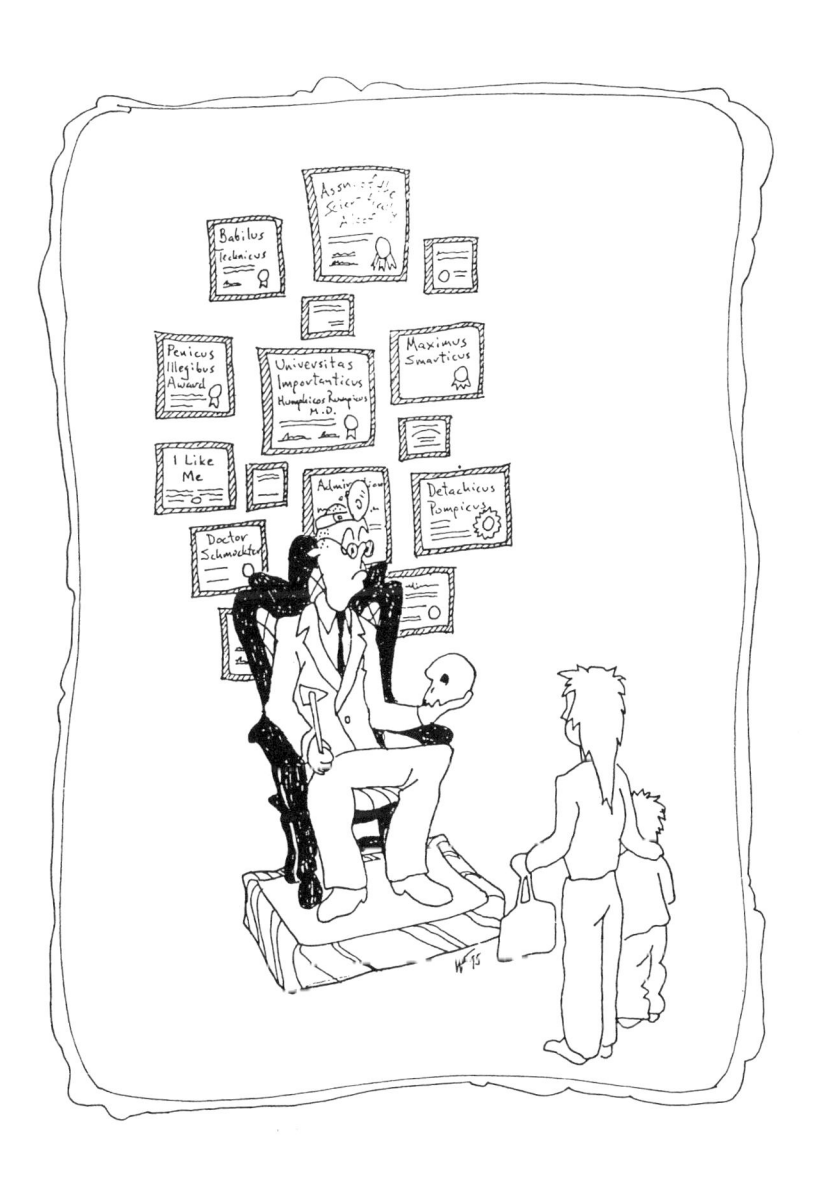

Such physicians will very seldom admit to their ignorance when unable to explain undiagnosed symptoms or lack of response to a given treatment. In those circumstances they may choose to order additional laboratory tests, no matter the expense, instead of resorting to consultation with a specialist. They tend to dismiss key observations made by patients regarding their clinical condition or effects of the treatment given. This can be easily explained by their strong need to take credit for positive outcomes.

Patients usually feel intimidated by physicians with narcissistic personality traits since they do not feel that their needs are being addressed in a caring and considerate manner.

Passive-Aggressive Personality Traits

Physicians with these traits have difficulties handling situations that involve negative feelings. They may not be able to take control when dealing with demanding patients and can be easily manipulated into scenarios where they are not following proper medical ethics. They also have a tendency to procrastinate in making important decisions regarding treatment, placing themselves at risk of malpractice on the basis of medical neglect.

These doctors do poorly when placed in positions of leadership or having to set limits. A good example is the doctor's incapacity to stand by his principles whenever he faces a hospital administrator's request which is really against the best interest of his patients.

Physicians with passive-aggressive personality traits are easily recognized by manipulative or antisocial patients who wish to get special treatment. Due to their difficulties setting limits and inability "to say no," they can end up prescribing controlled drugs to substance abusers who show up at their offices telling "sad stories." These are doctors who can be manipulated into providing inappropriate treatment to friends, acquaintances or co-workers.

They can also be exploited by fellow physicians when it is time to decide who will work double duty or cover for another medical worker during vacation time. The exception to this rule comes about when a doctor shows very marked passive-aggressive traits. In this case, he or she will be purposefully inefficient while covering for a colleague. Therefore, fellow doctors will know that it is risky to leave their patients under such physician's care.

Histrionic Personality Traits

Physicians with these personality features tend to become involved in self-dramatization and have a strong need to draw attention to themselves. These doctors are the ones who would spend an inordinate amount of time during an office visit telling the patient about their own personal experiences. Patients have serious difficulties communicating with these doctors, since they feel ignored and very much placed in a secondary role.

Doctor-Patient Relationship

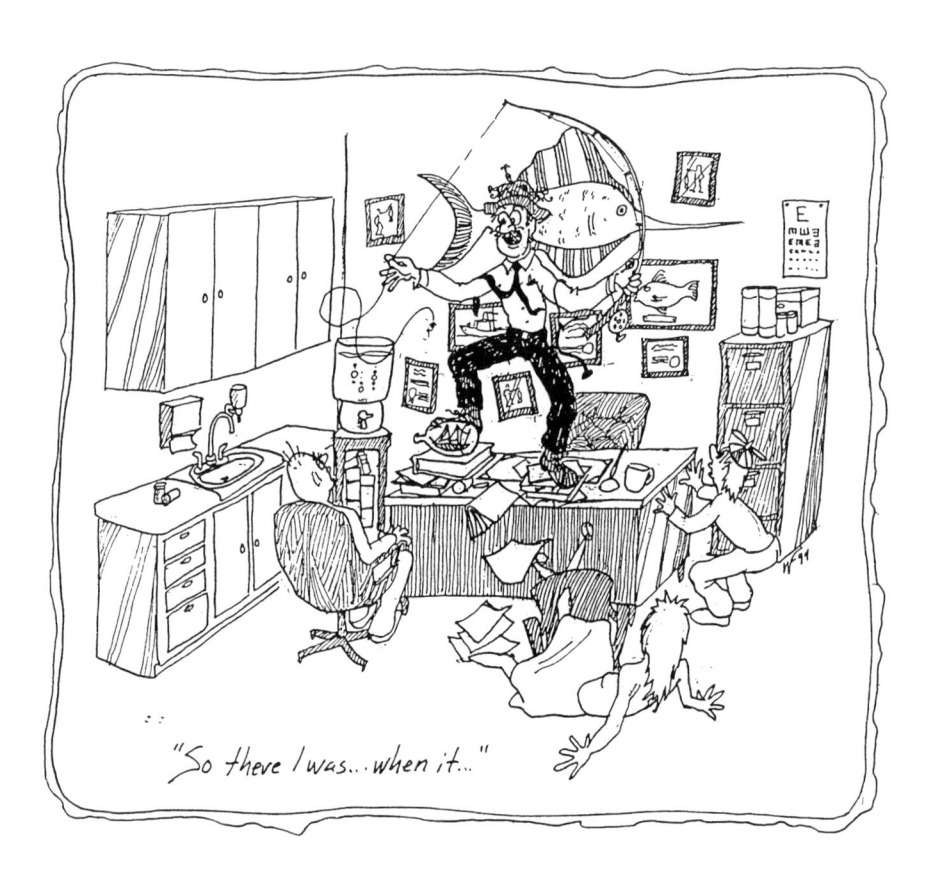

"So there I was...when it..."

Physicians with histrionic tendencies are also prone to overreact to minor events and may throw temper tantrums in front of patients and co-workers. In general, they are egocentric, self-indulgent and often inconsiderate of others. As a consequence they can be perceived as shallow and lacking genuineness. Additionally, they have the propensity to be demanding and overtly critical. This hampers their ability to relate to patients in an objective and caring manner.

These characteristics definitely affect their job performance, since they often lack insight and do poorly in regards to self-evaluation. They do better when they have special skills in technical areas and when they count on supervisors who are flexible and supportive.

Antisocial Personality Traits

Physicians with these traits lack moral standards. They often display unlawful behavior involving criminal mischief during adolescence, with chronic violation of rules at home and school. Their personal lives many times are complicated by physical assaults on family members, sexual promiscuity, failure to honor financial obligations, substance abuse and the tendency to be unfaithful to their spouses.

Many of these doctors end up having their medical licenses revoked due to violation of the standards of medical ethics. As a consequence, they move around the country, specially those affected by alcohol and/or drug abuse.

Naive patients can be easy preys of these doctors because most individuals with antisocial tendencies often present themselves to others as "charming." Therefore, it will be natural for many clients to place their full trust on such physicians without realizing that they are unethical.

Schizoid Personality Traits

Physicians with these personality features usually choose to go into medical specialties such as pathology, research or radiology, which require minimal direct contact with patients.

These medical workers may be impaired in their capacity to socialize and tend to be indifferent to the feelings of others. They come across as being detached from their environment and are frequently absent-minded. In addition, they prefer to be alone and away from human contact.

Avoidant Personality Traits

Physicians with these personality characteristics are frequently affected by low self-esteem. They are also sensitive to rejection, humiliation and shame. These doctors tend to avoid social events and instead invest disproportionate amounts of time reading or conducting research projects.

Doctor-Patient Relationship 27

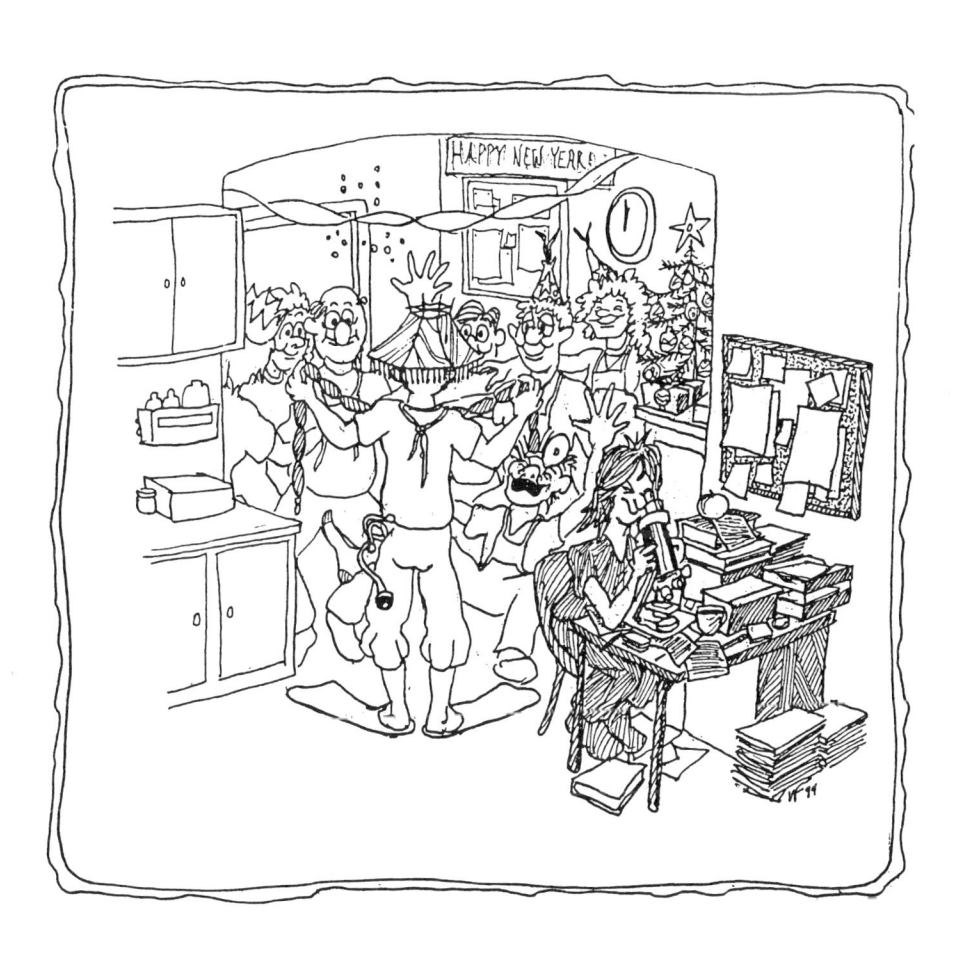

They differ from others with Schizoid Personality traits because they have a sincere need for approval. Despite their ability to establish closeness, these individuals do not risk personal involvement unless they feel accepted.

Physicians with avoidant personality features react poorly to professional success and tend to devaluate themselves, in spite of their obvious achievements.

Paranoid Personality Traits

These physicians have great difficulties working in institutions since they frequently question loyalty and expect trickery from others. They tend to be preoccupied with legal matters and spend an uncommon amount of time paying attention to malpractice issues. As a consequence of this, they distance themselves from the main objective, which is to maintain a positive relationship with the patient.

Doctors with paranoid personality characteristics are usually extremely serious and often are deprived of sentimental, soft and tender feelings. Because of this they are perceived by their patients as cold and unemotional.

Personality Disorders

Physicians affected by a personality disorder show exaggerated features from those presented in the previous pages. According to the DSM IV, Diagnostic and Statistical Manual of Mental Disorders, personality disorders are mani-

Doctor-Patient Relationship

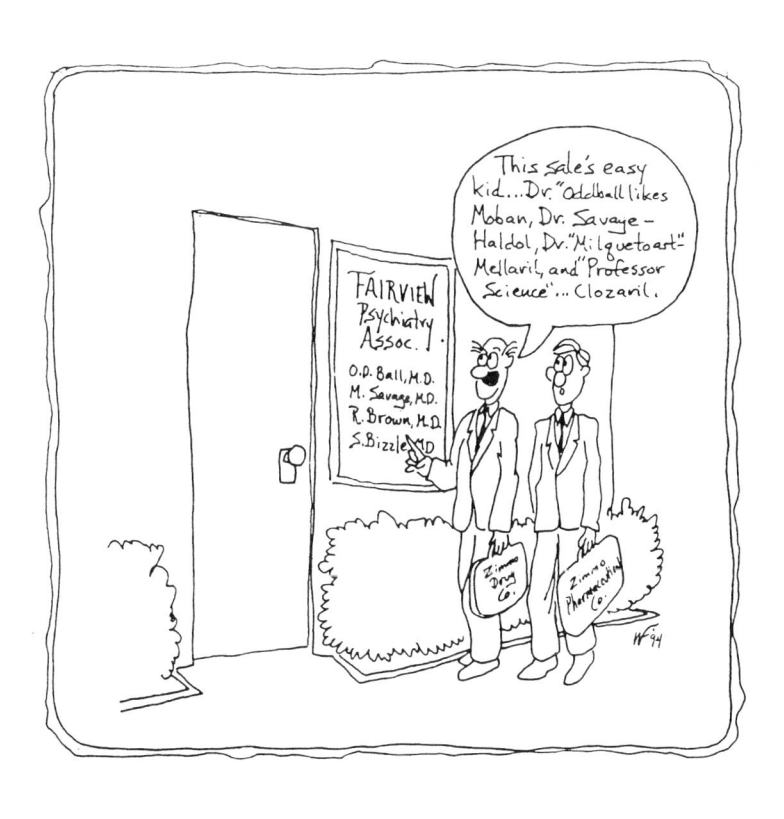

fested when a person shows evidence of personality traits which are "inflexible and maladaptive". This is the same to say that their lives are mainly ruled by their disorder, which generates behaviors that are detrimental to the patients and the medical community as well.

As a rule of thumb, one can very easily identify a person with this kind of impairment whenever he literally gets "under one's skin."

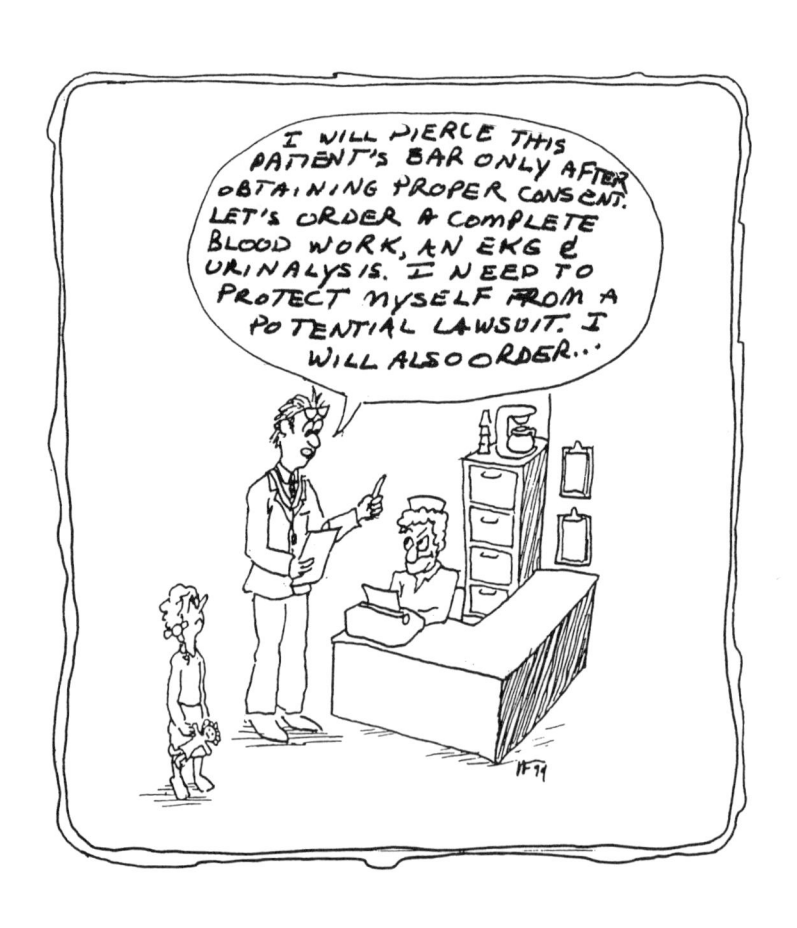

THE THREAT OF MALPRACTICE SUITS

In recent years there has been a great increase in the number of legal actions against physicians. Because of this, doctors are often concerned in rendering "the best of their services" in order to avoid the penalties related to medical malpractice. This leads to taking a good number of precautions to protect the doctor from the patient, who can be perceived as a potential adversary. In this scenario, the client can become that individual who at any time may sue the doctor. Such situation may prompt the doctor to deal with his client in a more mechanical way and with less spontaneity.

Physicians are then in danger of being over concerned about protecting themselves and their credibility. The patient can be displaced into a secondary level. Therefore, the doctor-patient relationship, which needs to be based on genuine trust and humanitarian love can become impersonal, cold, artificial and potentially hostile.

WORK OVERLOAD AND STRESS

Physicians are a high risk group for the burnout syndrome. The main symptoms of this condition are feelings of emotional and physical exhaustion. In addition, there is a tendency to become detached from people and make negative remarks about patients. Other characteristics of burnout are frequent colds, decreased effectiveness of the immune system, marital conflicts, irritability and lack of enthusiasm in meetings.

It is, therefore, of prime importance that physicians familiarize themselves with the burnout syndrome in order to avoid suffering it. Factors that lead to this condition are among the following: work overload, contact with chronic or terminally ill patients, lack of hobbies or recreational activities and family conflicts. Doctors who are idealistic are more predisposed to experience burnout, since they have high expectations about the outcome of treatment.

Physicians experiencing burnout may come across as distant and uninvolved. When this is the case, they tend to act in a mechanical way and will show an apparent lack of interest in the well-being of others. Patients may misinterpret this behavior as a sign of rejection, believing that the doctor is indifferent and unconcerned about them.

Doctor-Patient Relationship

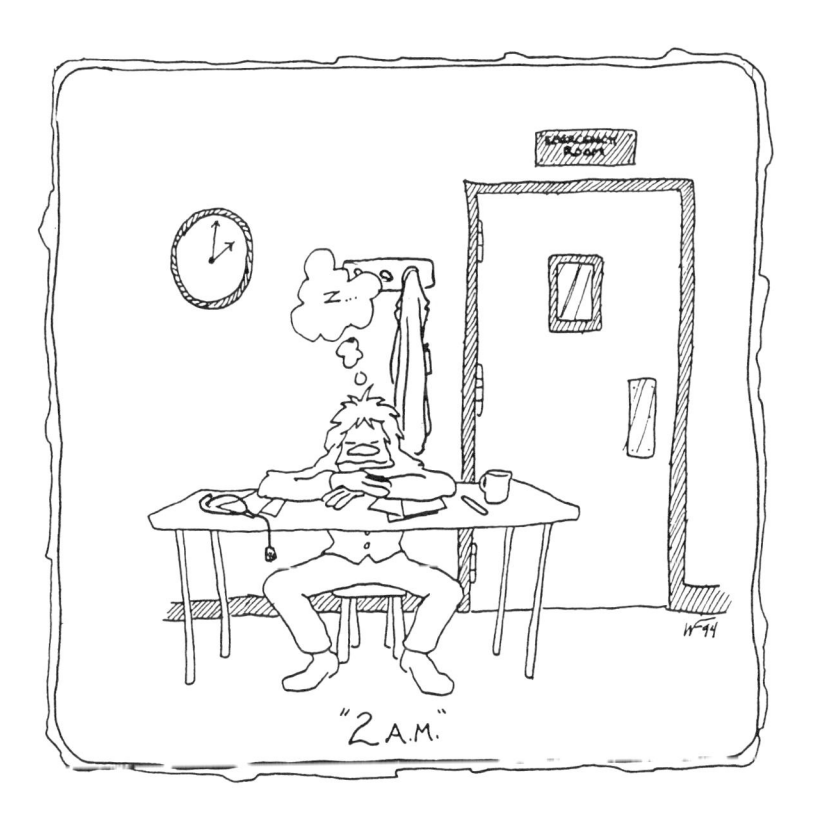

It appears that there is an unspoken tradition among doctors that it is appropriate for them to work long uninterrupted hours. It is routine in hospitals for a physician to be expected to return to a full day of work, following a 36 hour shift of O.D. duty. This attitude puts them in the position of being "crusaders" and always ready to sacrifice their health, as they strive in emulating altruistic needs. Many physicians find themselves forced to use different means to stay awake during night duty. They do so through drinking large amounts of coffee, smoking cigarettes and even resorting to illegal use of psychostimulants.

The role of the physician as a "service provider" and not "a care taker" needs to be reviewed in order to prevent more medical workers from falling into the path of burnout.

THE PHYSICIAN'S UNCONSCIOUS FEELINGS

The patient's feelings towards the doctor are a common source of "resistance" in complying with the prescribed treatment. The client not only reacts to who the physician is, but also to what the doctor symbolizes in the patient's unconscious world. The patient tends to displace to the doctor feelings which were first experienced for persons who played an important role during his or her childhood.

In technical terms, this is the transference mechanism that occurs in all relationships. It is more frequently directed to those who represent authority, which is generally the case with the physician. Therefore, many patients can easily transfer to the doctor feelings that were previously experienced towards the first authority figures in their lives: their parents or surrogate parents.

From the physician's side, there are also barriers that affect his behavior when interacting with some patients. This occurs whenever a patient's behavior awakens feelings in the doctor's unconscious, related to the ones previously experienced during his early life. When physicians are unaware of this reaction, called countertransference, they may have difficulties in their relationship with specific patients. Therefore, they may behave in a somewhat distant or even hostile manner, despite being accurate in their technique. However, when aware of these dynamics, the doctor can constructively utilize his anxiety or the negative feelings aroused from this relationship to assist the patient in profiting from treatment.

The transference/countertransference phenomenon can be illustrated in the following schematic diagram :

DOCTOR	PATIENT
POSITIVE COUNTER TRANSFERENCE	**POSITIVE TRANFERENCE**
Eager to see the patient	Desire to please the physician
Feeling positive when in his or her presence	Cooperative behavior with treatment
Willingness to invest on the patient	Need for the doctor's approval

DOCTOR	PATIENT
NEGATIVE COUNTER TRANSFERENCE	**NEGATIVE TRANSFERENCE**
Unexplained uneasiness facing the patient	Oppositional behavior toward treatment
Lack of investment on the given patient	Resistance to comply with treatment
A particular dislike for the patient	Withholding important information

The doctors main duty as a potential healer is to utilize all the sources available to activate or release the healing process in the patient. Often the patient expects to be healed or at least to obtain some benefits from a given treatment. This is not always attainable.

In many of these situations the physician faces an oppositional patient whose unconscious attitude is expressed by signs such as:

- Difficulties in keeping appointments or showing up late.
- Failure to take the prescribed medication or taking it in an incorrect way.
- Lack of motivation in following diets, exercise programs and specific medical recommendations.
- Resistance in changing behaviors and attitudes that are detrimental to the good quality of his or her life.

The physician must be prepared to deal with manifestations of non-compliance by the patient, which may have conscious or unconscious motivation. The doctor needs to be willing to help the client to change his negative attitude. In this situation it is important that he spend more time with the patient who is engaged in sabotaging the treatment process.

To help the patient to become more cooperative, the physician's number one priority is to establish the best level of communication. The most productive interaction between these two people is one that is based on an atmosphere of universal love, trust and mutual cooperation.

The association between doctors and patients is a partnership in which physicians are "selling their expertise" to benefit those who seek to be cured, or at least alleviated from their distress, illness or unbalanced condition. If the medical professional delivers the therapeutic message in an appropriate technical fashion, but with a rejecting or unfriendly manner, the patient will show signs of non-compliance. Then, the client in an overt or hidden fashion will oppose the treatment even though he or she knows it is the correct approach to assist the doctor in treating the disorder.

It is unusual for medical doctors to think of themselves as the ones who can block the good results of a given treatment, or cause the patient to become resistant in cooperating. In fact, it seems paradoxical to say that there are physicians who obstruct treatment. However, this happens, whenever the unconscious hostility and animosity that they harbor towards their patients do not allow them to succeed in rendering good professional care. Here, they are experiencing what can be called "self-sabotage."

Those physicians are in general sincerely committed to their clients, even though at an unconscious level they manage to undermine the results of their job. Therefore, in one way or another, they are perceived by the person in treatment as rejecting or hostile. The patient, then, gets the feeling of being betrayed and treated as a number and not as a human being.

These are some of the ways physicians may sabotage the treatment process:

1. Scheduling more patients than they can honestly handle. By doing so, they avoid spending quality time with each patient. Those treated by these physicians many times refer to the office as a "meat market."

2. Not focusing on the patient during consultation and instead being preoccupied with other issues. At times, they are concerned mostly about completing this consultation, in order to make time to see the next patient.

3. Being too technical and mechanical during interaction with the patient, especially when it is time to explain procedures.

4. Avoiding eye contact or using negative body language.

On the other hand, physicians can have a paternal attitude towards their clients. In this case, their behavior can take different forms such as permissive, punitive, critical or demanding. These distorted attitudes need to be replaced by a more appropriate behavior that can be aimed to benefit the patient and obtain better results from the treatment.

THE PHYSICIAN'S OWN HEALTH PROBLEMS

Most people have unrealistic expectations about physicians, believing that they are not supposed to become ill. This is a false concept. In reality there is a large population of "impaired physicians," who are in need of specialized treatment. In recent years, the medical community has become increasingly aware of this issue and so created organizations which offer help and support to doctors who are unable to meet standards of medical care because of health problems.

Impaired Physician's Societies now exist in many locations across the country. Members of these organizations provide support and assistance for impaired physicians.

These groups are connected with the State Board of Medical Examiners, as well as Alcoholic Anonymous and Narcotic Anonymous. They strongly urge impaired physicians to seek active treatment and are firm in their recommendations. They also monitor urine drug screens and specify the duration of specialized treatment. Officers of the Impaired Physician's Society are involved with medical schools, giving talks to the students. The Talbot Recovery Center in Atlanta, Georgia, is one of the main specialized centers for inpatient treatment dedicated to serve physicians suffering from substance abuse.

The following are the most frequent health problems affecting physicians:

Substance Abuse

The term substance abuse encompasses alcohol and drug abuse. Impaired Physician's Societies offer a variety of services to doctors who are experiencing problems with substance abuse. To more appropriately be of assistance to those physicians, the name of the Society has been proposed to change to "Physicians in Recovery." This is a welcomed effort to minimize the stigma of drug abuse and alcoholism among medical doctors.

In addition to this, in many cities, Veterinarians, Dentists and Psychologists, who are also in treatment for substance abuse are welcomed in joining the local Impaired Physician's Society.

Alcohol Abuse and Dependence

Dynamically speaking, alcoholics are detained at the oral stage of psychological development. Being fixated at this stage, they use the mouth as a vehicle to relieve anxiety and frustration. These individuals attempt to repress their anxiety, depression, sense of inadequacy, loneliness and other undesirable states of mind through drinking or abusing controlled drugs.

Physicians have difficulties recovering from alcohol abuse due to the nature of their work dealing on a daily basis with the pain and anxiety of their patients. Because of the importance of this issue it needs to be addressed whenever detected, especially during medical school.

Doctors who abuse alcohol, like any other person, can be affected by psychological distress and serious medical problems. As a result, they are susceptible to experiencing difficulties interacting with family members, peers, people in general and patients.

Those physicians abusing alcohol or drugs, who are not in treatment, are socially and occupationally impaired.

Narcotics Abuse and Dependence

The dynamics here are similar to those in alcohol abuse. Often, a problem with narcotics abuse or dependence will arise following an illness that requires temporary prescription of controlled drugs. This is the case with back injuries, kidney stones or any condition that causes severe physical pain. What complicates the picture is the fact that physicians have immediate access to controlled drugs, such as benzodiazepines, pain killers and others.

Cocaine Abuse

The actual incidence of cocaine abuse among physicians

is not known, since a good number of doctors who are cocaine abusers do not come to the attention of the Impaired Physician's Society. This is due to the fact that many of these doctors can still perform adequately at work in spite of using such drug. Because cocaine is a stimulant, the physician who abuses it will experience difficulties dealing with patients and co-workers due to sudden mood swings. When the cocaine abuse becomes more severe, the abuser will display symptoms of paranoia. Then, the doctor in question must be immediately assisted to commit himself to treatment.

Amphetamines Abuse and Dependence

Amphetamines abuse is more prevalent among medical students, interns and residents due to their need to stay up late, studying or performing night duties. When it becomes severe, it can lead into drug induced psychosis, with the presence of paranoid delusional thinking.

Cannabis Abuse

Cannabis abuse is also more frequent among medical students because of their exposure to the college culture. There are some who sponsor the legalization of marihuana. Such information may give young physicians the false idea that they will not be liable if they use this drug during hours of duty. However, it is well known that marihuana impairs a person's ability to think clearly and to perform technical procedures. This will increase the chances of human error in medical practice.

Physicians with substance abuse are more vulnerable to the self-destructive aspects of their illnesses because of the demanding nature of their occupation. Most of the time it is a tremendous burden for them to give support to the insecure, anxious or depressed patient, when in reality it is the doctor who is the one in great need for nurturance, reassurance and support.

It is mandatory for doctors to help the patients go through their battle against disease. For impaired physicians this becomes an overwhelming task, after they have been weakened by their own distress. By being handicapped, they are more qualified to receive support than to give it.

Physicians with HIV or AIDS

This is a whole new area where the American Medical Association and the Surgeon General have made definite recommendations. At this juncture, physicians who are HIV positive are not required to inform patients about their condition, unless they intend to perform "exposure prone procedures." The same principle applies to Hepatitis B infected physicians. In most states there are expert review panels that will advice the HIV/HBV-positive physician about in which circumstances he or she may need to disclose this information to patients.

The basic rule is to have the HIV-positive physician reviewed by an expert panel; and obtain informed consent from the patient prior to performing invasive procedures.

The American Medical Association is against requiring mandatory HIV testing as a condition to grant medical staff privileges. The Federation of State Medical Boards recommends the observation of the following policies by each State Medical Board:

1. Require that physicians performing exposure prone procedures know their HIV and HBV status.
2. Have the power to require reporting of HIV and HBV infected physicians by hospitals, clinics, etc.
3. Ensure the confidentiality of HIV and HBV infected physicians.
4. Establish practice guidelines for HIV and HBV infected physicians.
5. Monitor the practices of HIV and HBV infected physicians.
6. Discipline HIV and HBV infected physicians who violate laws preventing transmission of these viruses to patients.

Employers have the right to request HIV testing from health care workers who are considered to be a "significant threat" to the health of others. Therefore, if the hospital has a reasonable cause to believe that a physician may be HIV infected, that physician can be requested to reveal the results of his or her HIV testing.

Physicians affected by Mental Disorders

Whenever physicians experiences impairment in their ability to deliver care due to a mental disorder, they are required by the local State Medical Board to participate in treatment. Additionally, they must report to the appropriate medical authorities periodically. Doctors affected by these disorders are not addressed by the Impaired Physician's Society, which mainly assists those who abuse alcohol and controlled drugs. Therefore, these doctors cannot count on an organized support system. They are frequently ostracized by the medical staff of a given hospital.

It is of great importance that local chapters of the Impaired Physician's Society develop systems to provide adequate support and assistance for this group of doctors.

Physicians Suffering from Depression

There is a large number of medical doctors facing different degrees of depression. These physicians may experience serious economical set backs, since their productivity decreases significantly during episodes of depression. Whenever possible, they should switch to a medical specialty that is less demanding or stressful.

Fortunately, the treatment of this condition nowadays is fairly effective due to the availability of a variety of antidepressant medications. Depressed physicians should also pay attention to the location where they choose to live, especially if being affected by "Seasonal Affective Disorder." When this is the case, it is recommended to avoid setting up practice in northern states because of the long winters. Additionally, it is also important for them to stay away from specialties that deal with patients suffering from chronic illnesses or who are dying.

Physicians Affected by Bipolar Disorder

Physicians affected by bipolar disorder are manic-depressives. These cases are not rare because of the high incidence of this condition and the fact that many manic-depressives are high achievers. Doctors affected by bipolar disorder may go for several months without experiencing severe mood swings. Therefore, they may have a "normal" medical practice during those periods of time. However, when subjected to an episode of mania or depression, they will be temporarily unable to work. In this situation, it would be appropriate to take a leave of absence.

Due to the potential complications of bipolar disorder, physicians affected by it do better when working in a group, or for a large medical organization.

Those who are affected by this condition may experience buying sprees during episodes of mania. It is best for them not to carry credit cards and have a responsible and totally trusting family member, a spouse for instance, monitoring their finances. In addition, they should be encouraged to keep a substantial savings account and obtain disability health insurance.

It is recommended to all parties involved that whenever a physician shows deficiencies in his work performance, he should be first reported to the local Impaired Physician's Society. This is a more appropriate choice than resorting to the Board of Medical Examiners. Therefore, the Impaired Physician's Society is the initial step because of its level of understanding about the needs of a medical professional who faces health problems. This society seeks avenues that can prevent restrictions in medical practice by special mandates of the Board.

Hypochondriasis and Anxiety Disorders

According to the DSM IV, the main feature of hypochondriasis is "an unrealistic interpretation of physical signs or sensations as abnormal, leading to preoccupation with the fear or belief of having a serious disease."

There is a good percentage of physicians who can be considered hypochondriacs. This is the case with doctors who have high anxiety level and a tendency to develop panic attacks. They have great hardship going through medical school as they easily experience imaginary symptoms of many diseases when learning about them.

Anxiety, depressed mood and compulsive personality traits are common among these individuals. As a consequence, they are less able to offer reassurance to their patients when needed. These professionals may be impaired in their ability to deliver appropriate medical care because of excessive preoccupation with their own symptoms.

Overanxious physicians are prone to develop psychosomatic symptomatology. Therefore, it is recommended that they commit themselves to psychotherapy, in order to reach an improved level of control over their own anxiety.

Sexual Disorders

The incidence of sexual disorders among medical doctors is unknown due to the secrecy involved in the life style of individuals with these disorders. However, it is not infrequent to learn about physicians who are facing charges for sexual misconduct with their clients. Patients are easy targets to be sexually abused by physicians because they perceive the doctor as an omnipotent and powerful figure.

Doctors with problems in this area need close monitoring by medical authorities, since it is well known that treatment of sexual disorders is quite difficult, with a high percentage of recidivism.

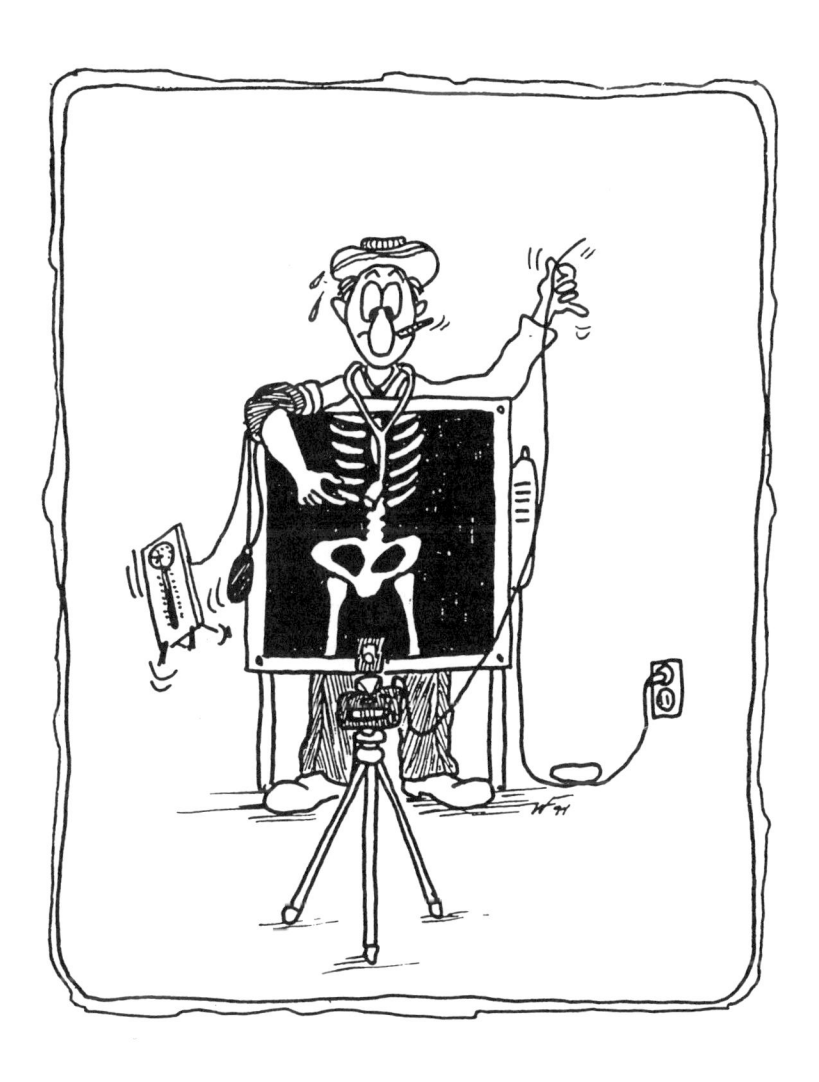

Doctor-Patient Relationship

THE EMERGENCY ROOM PHYSICIAN

The work performed by the emergency room doctor is extremely stressful because of its particular nature. It demands a great deal of energy, self-confidence, capacity to make decisions, compassion and high level of respect for human life.

In this particular situation, the doctor-patient relationship has a different connotation, considering that it does not follow the ordinary path of the interaction that takes place on a daily basis at the physician's office.

During this accelerated contact, there is limited time to develop the same quality of rapport as the one experienced by the members of other specialties and their patients. It is established when the patient may be facing a life threatening situation or attempting to cope with a severe physical-emotional pain or discomfort. This is the moment when a great degree of anxiety is mobilized, not only from the patient's side, but also from the physician's as well.

Sometimes the disorder presented by the patient is temporarily or permanently incapacitating, even fatal. It is necessary to understand why the sick individual is often destabilized, irrational, uncooperative, hostile, irritable or demanding, by the occasion of his or her visit to the Emergency Unit.

Physicians faced with this hard work have to be technically well trained, above all, stable, tolerant and compassionate. They also need to comprehend that a patient in such circumstances is mainly directed by feelings of fear and so incapable of exerting good judgment. Here, again, the doctor's number one concern must be the well-being of the one in treatment. It is crucial for physicians to be aware of the responsibility of their mission as mediators between the tangible and the intangible. While being conscientious about the fact that the outcome of the medical or surgical procedures lies in their hands, physicians must be eager to hold their emotions under positive control.

With this constructive frame of mind, doctors are able to put themselves in a position to treat their patients more successfully, or at least to comfort them with a level of compassion. This does not mean that developing this special type of attitude is an easy task. On the contrary! It seems to be one of the hardest positions in the medical field. Even so, it can be accomplished by those who really see the patient as a primary cause of the medical work. The results of such an excellent way of rendering services are highly rewarding. It is indeed most gratifying, despite being very stressful. Therefore, it is worthy to sacrifice oneself and spend quality energy while carrying on this mission.

THE DOCTOR'S PROFESSIONAL AND DOMESTIC LIFE

It is extremely hard to combine a successful professional life with a well adjusted interaction with one's own family. It requires a great deal of self-discipline, emotional balance and even physical health to develop and express good marital and parental skills, along with productive and rewarding work activity.

It seems that this problem affects any person who faces a demanding life, especially medical doctors with the peculiarities of their occupation. The challenge is more overwhelming if the physician is a female who happens to be a mother and a wife. Her limited time needs to be well managed to assist and nurture her family, while providing responsible and loving care to her patients.

The male doctor can be overloaded by his stressful job and responsibilities as a father and a husband, as well. It is easy for him to be caught up by the pressure and demands of his work. In such a situation, family life is sacrificed in favor of his medical duties.

Sometimes, the spouses and the children are neglected

Doctor-Patient Relationship

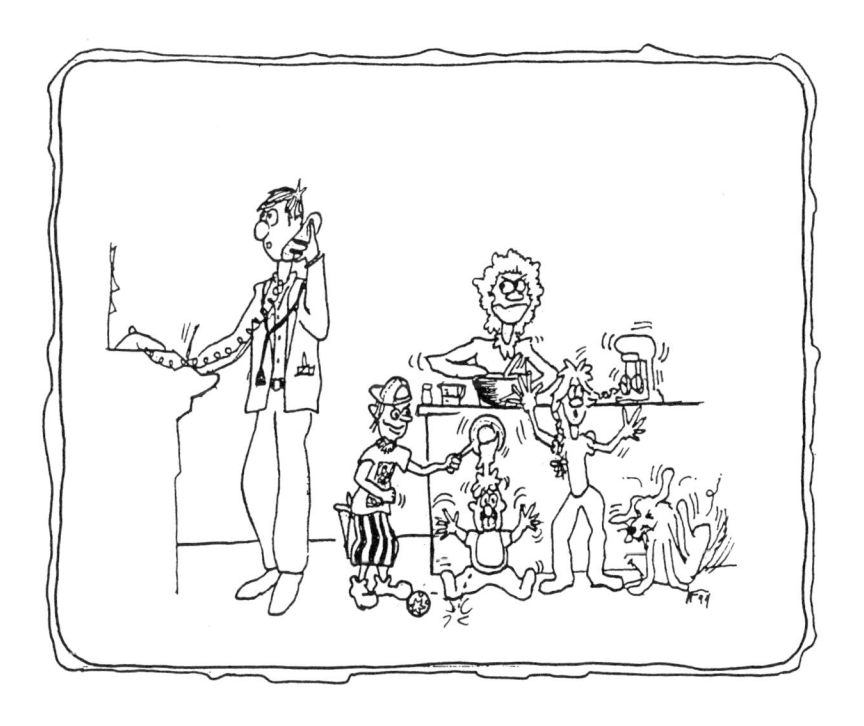

because there is no quality time available for them. This generates a sense of alienation between the stressed physician and his or her family. The spouse and the children feel deprived of the bright and successful doctor who is their father, mother, husband or wife. As a consequence, there is a breakdown in their relationship and both sides try to deal with the pain generated by this sense of emptiness, by retreating into fear, anger, guilt and mutual self-punishment. The physician who suffers this pressure on his domestic relationships does not have the internal peace to run his life, either as a family person, or as a professional worker.

The doctor, like any other individual in society, emerges from different types of social settings, ranging from well adjusted to very dysfunctional ones. Whenever the physician's early years were marked by discord, hostility and poor expression of love among family members, they will face more difficulties in their domestic and professional life.

Many negative experiences could have affected physicians during their childhood, including several varieties of sick parenting. Sometimes, the physician was an object of neglectful, cold, or hostile parents. In other occasions, the parents were alcoholics, drug abusers, or even mentally ill.

After being exposed to these types of stressors, the medical doctor will be less able to accomplish quality work with patients. At the same time, his or her ability to be an effective parent and caring spouse will be impaired. The outcome is frequently about the same: an anxious doctor trying to cope with his own maladjusted family. This may result in marital discord, divorce, substance abuse, misconduct, or other expressions of unbalanced life in all the persons involved.

In the preceding pages of this book one has seen a number of problems that can impair physicians and prevent them from reaching their full potential. No matter what the reason of their distress, there are several ways to help the afflicted doctors to respond in a healthier manner to the demands of their lives.

What is described above is not what always happens in the physician's world. There are also those who have the ability to manage their professional and domestic lives well. In these cases no one will be deprived of the doctor's best care. When this is possible, the doctor is fulfilling the position that society expects from him or her as a positive role model.

But what happens when this is not the case? Here, there is an important question: What one should do to prevent the doctor's private life from becoming unmanageable and his or her work activities from turning into an uncontrollable roller coaster? There are many ways to reestablish the balance that one has lost, no matter what is the cause. Relaxation, stress management techniques, counseling, conventional and unconventional psychotherapeutic approaches can be of great help, as well as meditation and yoga.

In recent years, increased attention has been paid to the quality of life of physicians. Workshops and seminars are now available for doctors and spouses, in order for them to work on issues related to their family life. For those who are insightful enough to recognize the necessity of this personal effort, the benefits are unquestionable. The Menninger Foundation, in Topeka Kansas, is well known for its expertise in this area.

ETHICAL BOUNDARIES

Economical, Social and Sexual Involvement with Patients

From the ethical point of view, there are aspects of the doctor-patient relationship that contribute to lower the high standards on which this partnership should be based. This can occur when the doctor uses the patient as an instrument of social involvement, financial gain or an object of erotic feelings.

Doing business or socializing with a client, outside of the professional setting is absolutely unethical. Even so, this is not unusual among family doctors, or others outside of the psychiatric field. Psychiatrists are the only medical workers who have been warned against this practice.

In small communities, where doctors have more opportunities to get closer to their patients and vice-versa, the breach of the ethical boundaries occurs more frequently. Here, the concern of the authors is mainly directed to doctors' sexual indiscretions with their patients.

Through the years, the sexual involvement by clients with psychiatrists, psychologists, and other mental health pro-

Doctor-Patient Relationship

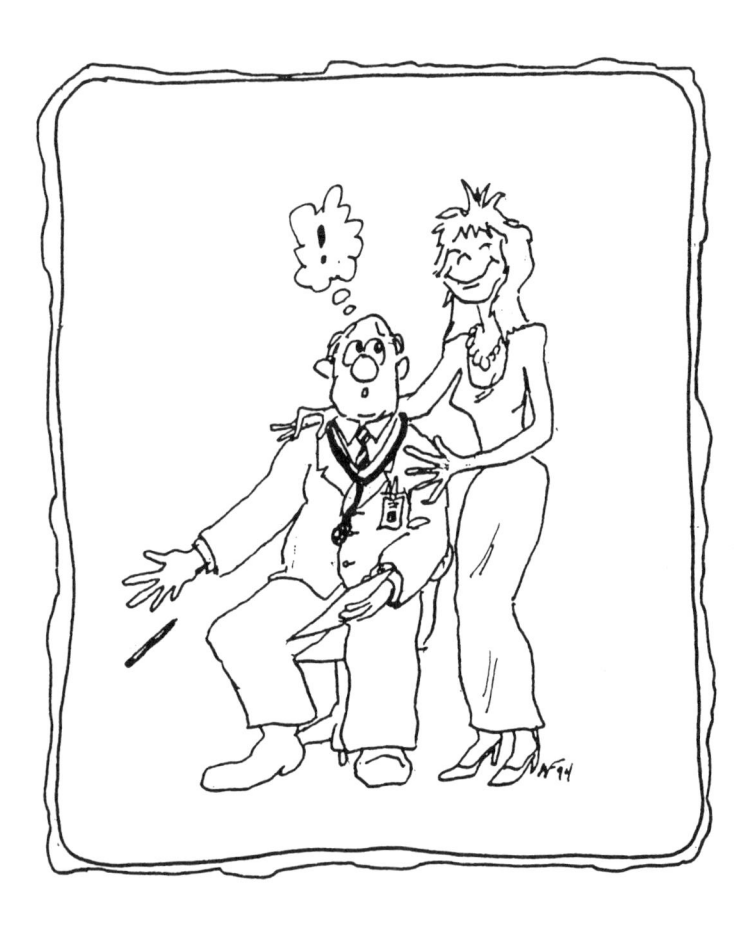

Doctor-Patient Relationship

fessionals has been an object of serious attention by the medical and legal systems. However, only after the seventies have such erotic behaviors been more openly discussed by society and among physicians as well. These reports have demonstrated that primary care physicians also use their patients as sexual objects.

Fortunately, during recent years more cases are coming to the public eye as a consequence of legal action by the victims of such abuse. Indeed, in the past. not so many people felt encouraged to come forward and disclose being molested by the respectable person in charge of their health care. This is gradually changing as society is more aware about its prerogatives and less intimidated by the figure of the " All Powerful Doctor."

Lately, with the increasing number of documented cases of sexual misconduct by doctors inside and outside the psychiatric field, the American Medical Association has established ethical guidelines addressing this relevant issue.

Statistically speaking, there are variations in prevalence regarding the medical specialty involved. However, there is no real exception for any particular medical area when it is time to focus on this sensitive matter.

Apparently, the breach on this sacred relationship has taken place since immemorial times, considering the admonition expressed in the Hippocratic Oath: "I will come for the benefit of the sick, remaining free of all intentional injustice, of all mischief and in particular of sexual relationship with both female and male persons, be they free or slaves."

In many States, it is expressly illegal for mental health doctors to be engaged in sexual activities with any one under their professional care. So far, the legislation is only directed to the workers in the mental health area and does not include physicians from other specialties who have sexually victimized their patients. It seems that the patient's dignity continues to be increasingly violated through the sexual advances of their doctors, despite the fact that this is explicitly forbidden under the ethical-legal-social perspective.

Furthermore, it is not rare that opposite situations also occur. This is when the physician is the target of seductive patients, who cross the moral line between themselves and their physicians. In these cases, the patient tries and often succeeds in getting romantically involved with the doctor. To be able to stop patients from getting them involved in sexual intimacy, medical doctors must hold a strong conviction of their ethical-professional values and be emotionally stable. Through this behavior they will help patients to keep appropriate moral boundaries towards them .

Considering the attraction which may be felt by the physician, when the patient makes romantic advances, many times it is not easy for him or her to prevent the lowering of the moral standards of the doctor-patient relationship. Here, the medical worker must firmly reject any attempt by the client to destroy the special bond, even if he may have to dismiss the patient.

The attraction that is felt by the patient towards the doctor and the erotic feelings experienced in the opposite direction should be viewed as transference and countertransference. Dynamically speaking, the physician represents to the client a similar role as the parental figures do, holding both a position that has a dimension of authority along with a caregiving responsibility. On the client's side there can be a pattern of dependence and vulnerability that needs to be respected at any price. Therefore, no physician should use his or her authority to deprive a person of a reliable source of emotional-physical healing through this unacceptable conduct.

Unconscious unresolved issues from the early days of the patient's life, and the doctor's as well, may lead them to be mutually engaged in erotic behaviors. Acting out sexual feelings, instead of translating them into verbal language, can be interpreted as an expression of resistance, very often used by the patient to obstruct the psychotherapeutic process. The mechanism of resistance is most apparent during psychotherapy. However, it can be detected in any other medical encounter. The patient may show different forms of resistance by opposing the physician's efforts to fight the disease. This should be brought to the patient's conscious level, in order for the treatment to be successful.

The emotional scars on patients who are sexually involved with primary care physicians or psychiatrists are similar in their deleterious results.

From a dynamic point of view, one can say that those emotions expressed or not in treatment by he patient towards the doctor are basically directed to what the physician represents in the client's unconscious world. The same phenomenon can be applied to the medical workers when clients awakens in them unconscious feelings that were first experienced by them in their childhood. Therefore, nothing is indeed related to the doctor's, or to the client's appearance, sex appeal or attractiveness. Anyone who happens to become romantically involved in this setting would be expressing "vicarious" feelings that otherwise would be addressed to the important figures of his past.

In conclusion, any attitude or behavior that can contribute to jeopardize the healthy interaction between doctor and patient must be considered detrimental for both. As any other unethical act, it should be avoided and handled through all the sources available. A very helpful preventive measure would be to make these issues part of the curriculum of the medical schools.

Learning about moral values and how to stand by them, especially at the time when one begins his or her career, is highly beneficial to all the persons involved and to society as well. This is extremely helpful to prevent suffering and embarrassment for both sides. Furthermore, many unpleasant law suits would be avoided.

CONCLUSIONS

After reviewing a number of aspects of physicians' lives and how they relate to their clients, there are still important questions to be answered:

- What motivates people who choose to enter medical school?
- Why does one decide to spend so many years of hard training to become a physician?

It seems that there is a range of motives, conscious and unconscious, defining the medical field as a career choice. Those reasons may be based on idealistic purposes or on more superficial, irrelevant or pragmatic intentions. It is not unusual that a candidate for medical school may feel compelled by a conscious desire to help people in their struggle against diseases. In other situations, the prospective physician is mainly motivated by the wish to become financially prosperous, in order to have easier access to a comfortable material life. Social status and prestige can also be considered a priority.

Regardless the motivations that direct the future doctor towards his professional selection, he is at an unconscious level basically guided by the deeply rooted desire to serve and help the suffering person. Most of the time, however, the individual is not aware of the idealism that lies beyond any type of "practical or less altruistic" justification for him or her to become a medical doctor.

This being so, why are not some physicians able to give to their patients a more compassionate and loving treatment?

Why are these doctors so arrogant, unkind, cold or simply detached from those who are their clients and in a position to receive humanitarian and nurturing support?

The basic answer to this difficult question is that some physicians are only technically qualified for their jobs. This is the same as to say that, at an emotional level, they are in more need for help and compassion than the ones under their care.

Here it is crucial to use this opportunity to address a strong message to the medical community to REHUMANIZE its sacred mission. This means that it is indispensable to deliver UNIVERSAL LOVE, COMPASSION and UNDERSTANDING, along with the prescribed medical or surgical procedures.

Doctors who coldly interact with their clients are those who have difficulty in touching their own emotions and finding appropriate solutions for their internal conflicts. Sometimes, their problems are beyond the so-called dysfunctional behavior. Those professionals are victims of undisclosed psychiatric problems, which can range from mild to severe. Under these conditions, their communication with patients becomes most of the time difficult and uneasy.

As mentioned before in this book, the Society for Impaired Physicians, operating nationwide and in connection with state medical boards, is indeed a very valuable organization. However, it mainly assists those professionals who happen to be addicted to alcohol and/or controlled substances. In spite of being efficient and helpful in these areas, so far, it only covers a limited percentage of the medical population in need of assistance.

Considering the multiplicity of the pathological entities affecting M.D.s, in silence, a broader specialized network is necessary for helping impaired physicians to accept the reality of their own illnesses. Once the stage of denial is past, the difficulty in seeking medical attention as a mandatory solution is easier to be attained.

Unfortunately, doctors are not mutually supportive when facing challenges in their personal lives. On the contrary! Sometimes, they are even cruel and judgmental of each other. In other words, they tolerate poorly any kind of failure in their lives or the lives of their peers. Narcissistic features are a very common trait in physicians' personalities. These do not allow them to admit their own limitations and the frailties of their colleagues as human beings. It seems to be forgotten that they are subjected to the same physical, emotional and spiritual laws, as any other ordinary individual.

Some medical schools concentrate mainly in teaching their students about the mechanical work necessary in dealing with patients. This goes from the simple task of how to prescribe medication to the most technically sophisticated medical or surgical procedures. In those schools there is less concern about teaching how to understand patients and their feelings. In doing so, they fail to acknowledge the importance of emotions and how they can affect the client's health.

The message subliminally delivered here is that future doctors should not get close to their patients. It seems that there is a fear of being "too close" to the patients and their pain, with the false assumption that medical students would loose perspective on the work to be accomplished. Therefore, there is an unspoken rule that has been transmitted from generation to generation of doctors that "they should not be involved." This means that they must be detached from their patients and their painful life, in order to be more "technically effective."

This statement is stronger when it is used in the hospital setting by the medical team in referring, for example, to "a case of leukemia," on "the bed number 12." Sometimes, this allusion is made without even mentioning the patient's name, showing disregard for his physical discomfort and emotional pain. It seems that there is little concern about the occupant of that bed, who may be facing a life threatening situation. This attitude triggers negative feelings in the sick person, consequently worsening his physical health.

Interacting in this way with a patient is very dehumanizing because, by doing so, he or she is treated as an object, a machine, a number, whose identity is completely denied by the medical team. From all this, one could reach to the conclusion that physicians are to learn, to teach and to profit academically and financially, using the patient's body as a tool. When this is the case, the client's human, emotional and spiritual aspects are virtually ignored.

To illustrate this discussion, let us describe a typical example of poor communication between a doctor and his patient. This event took place at a specialized clinic. A patient was scheduled to undergo surgery to be performed by the chief of the staff. At the time of the operation, a member of the professional group, unknown to the patient, showed up and without introducing himself to the client, silently started preparing him for the surgery. No word was spoken to the frightened patient, who expected to be operated on by the physician with whom he had developed a long term relationship. At that point, the patient decided to break the silence. He greeted the surgeon who, at first, did not answer and could not listen to anything because he was too involved in "doing his job." For him the surgery was considered to be the important issue. His attention was entirely turned towards what he perceived to be the object of his professional care, that segment of the patient's body on which the operation was to occur.

What about the patient's feelings? What about his emotions, fears and difficulties at that scary moment?

This was not the part of the surgeon's immediate preoccupation! His concern appeared to be directed towards doing everything perfectly in the technical sense. He underestimated the important emotional aspects of the body he was operating on. He had forgotten the patient as a human being, with feelings and emotions, and not an inanimate machine to be repaired. The appropriate behavior in this case would have been for the first surgeon to inform the patient about changing places with his associate. Furthermore, the new physician should have introduced himself, before starting the surgical procedure.

It is of prime importance that doctors place themselves in the position of being a patient, in order to feel what is it like to be on the other side. This issue was clearly portrayed in the movie *The Doctor*.

The following is another example that illustrates the behavior of physicians who are poorly able to acknowledge the patient's emotional world: A certain physician was in charge of treating a foreign patient in a general hospital. The client did not speak or understand a single word of English. Another doctor, a member from the same staff, was invited to be the interpreter between the patient and the medical team. When the interpreter physician approached the sick man, he was told that he only had five minutes to interview the patient, a 22-year-old man who was in poor health and confined to a wheel chair, perhaps for the rest of his life. While the interpreter physician was trying to do his best, "in only five minutes," the head of the staff, one more time, showed his impatience, hostility and lack of concern for the suffering of that person, by saying: "You, doctor, should encourage him to speak English."

How could someone, in such poor health speak, even in his native language? How could he have motivation to initiate at this time his learning of a foreign language?

When talking about how feelings may influence the manifestations of an illness, it is important to call the reader's attention to the new spot in medical research, Psychoneuroimmunoloy. Through the studies connected to this area one can understand more clearly the interdependence between the immunological, neurological systems and the emotional realm. Stress, depression, repressed or unresolved anger, hostility and other negative states of mind may contribute to disrupt the immune system on its disease-fighting network. Therefore, in order to help the patient to regain health, the physician needs to look beyond the physical signs and symptoms. Therefore, he should concentrate in learning about what comes along with the expression of the patient's somatic problems. For instance, a physician can be treating a person who presents a clinical picture of a gastrointestinal disturbance. Many times, such condition is triggered by suppressed anger related to unresolved conflicts.

Of course, every individual experiences his unbalance, distress or uneasiness under a different constellation of features. For some reason, many may "choose" to present emotional symptoms when they face the challenges of their lives, while others "exit" through some segment of their physical body that is more prone to be broken down in its physiological organization. Based on this premise, one can conclude that physicians who mainly concentrate in "curing bodies," without exploring the emotional and spiritual aspects behind the nosological frames, are missing very important tools to be used in the battle against illnesses. This does not mean that one must be or should act as a psychiatrist to succeed in treating patients. In any specialty, the physician should be skillful enough to deal with his client as a whole being, constituted of spiritual, emotional and physical aspects.

The difficulty in managing their "precious" hours of work has often been rationalized as a good reason why the doctor does not spend enough time with each patient. The current justification for this behavior is that there is no enough available hours to adequately see all the scheduled clients. This is probably true if one considers the economical side as a first priority. But, if the patient is perceived as the special, unique or even sacred part of the physician's job, the material aspect of the medical work will take a secondary position. Then, the doctors may not benefit financially as much, however, the quality of their professional services will be upgraded.

RECOMMENDATIONS

During the process of communicating with the patient, the physician faces a paramount issue: to be attentive and listen to whatever the person may have to say. Most of the time, the sick individual needs to talk to the doctor about something that is always important, no matter how "irrelevant" it may be from the physician's point of view. However, the patient does not always feel encouraged by the physician to verbalize his or her thoughts.

A sensitive doctor will listen to the client and try to engage in a clear and objective dialogue. This is the time when the doctor has the opportunity to learn about the client as a person who has feelings, positive or negative, along with the signs and symptoms that define his ailments. Of course, everybody to a certain extent, experiences undesirable feelings. What needs to be evaluated is if those emotions are powerful enough to trigger the disease in question or to influence the degree of its expression. In order to better understand the influence of feelings in the patient's illness, the doctor needs to spend quality time with him. Only by doing so can the physician get to know the person who is behind the disease. This is perfectly acceptable if the doctor is conscious that his assignment is to treat human beings who may present a dysfunction in their body-mind-soul composition. Through this deeper interaction with the client, the physician gains insight about the patient's physical-emotional baggage.

When the physician and the patient work as a team, the client becomes aware that the medical treatment is not only the doctor's prerogative, but his as well. Therefore, listening attentively and rationally to the patient, gives to the doctor more opportunities to succeed in achieving the ultimate goal in this unique partnership. The person in treatment feels that he is also a dynamic figure, indispensable for the healing work and for the attainment of a higher quality of life.

The language used must be clear and in line with the patient's level of education and comprehension. Technical terminology is better understood by the lay person when translated into simple words. It is also more productive if the doctor does not hesitate to repeat his statements. Later, the physician should go through a double check whenever the patient shows an indication of doubt or lack of understanding about what is being shared. One must not forget that even simple matters "are not well understood" when they are related to health problems or something that is not working well physically or emotionally in one's life. This means that the subject is being unconsciously blocked because of the anxiety generated by the fear existing behind it.

Making good eye contact with the patient is also very

significant for the sake of this relationship and its positive therapeutic results. It is a sign that the doctor is not intimidated by the patient's presence and is not particularly anxious about his or her approval as an individual and professional. The discussion about the specific treatment plan, surgical procedures or other measures to be followed is better understood when it takes place in a relaxed atmosphere, such as the doctor's office, rather than in the examination room. Not to do so gives to the patient a message that the physician is always in a hurry or running late. This can raise the client's suspiciousness about being used as a simple object or to increase the doctor's financial status.

To act in a relaxed and self-confident fashion physicians need not to be afraid of expressing feelings, behaving as caring human beings and presenting themselves as authentic as possible. It is important for doctors to learn about what kind of individuals they are and to get acquainted with the positive and negative traits of their own personalities. When this is properly done, doctors have the opportunity to correct some of their own imperfections.

The more aware doctors are about who they are, the better will be the quality of their work.

It does not matter as much if physicians are using the most sophisticated type of machines, tools or techniques. It is crucial for the persons receiving the treatment to feel, before everything else, that the doctor in charge of taking care of their health is really concerned about their welfare.

To prove to society that the medical worker has outstanding skills must not be the primary preoccupation of the one who deals with the most precious "merchandise" on Earth, the life of a fellow being.

CLOSING THOUGHTS

After approaching the most significant aspects of the physician-patient relationship, it is relevant to close this book with the ideas that may be the base for improving the quality of this partnership. Doctors would get more positive therapeutic results if they deliberately spend more time with their patients. Ideally, the physician should personally take the medical history like in the old days. Then, they could learn, first hand, about the important events of the client's life. Along with the history comes the knowledge of feelings such as fear, anger, hostility and other negative and positive states of mind that make up the patient's world. This would be a good opportunity for the medical professionals and their patients to work together. In this fashion they will obtain the best results from the treatment to be delivered.

Many times, just by sharing the undesirable emotions hidden behind a syndrome, a psychosomatic manifestation or even "a typical" physiopathological process there is a resolution or at least a relieve of the condition.

It is important to remind the doctor that in some cases, the patient, unconsciously, may choose "to protest" against his emotions, failings, frustrations and unresolved conflicts. This can be done by "sickening" the body or a part of it that is more vulnerable. Therefore, by getting to know "the mysteries" that one holds in his emotional world, the physician has "an informative map" that will help the patient to unblock the path that leads to his own healing.

Then, the doctor has a unique opportunity to work as a facilitator for the restoration of the health process.

When the medical worker is able to walk with the patient, shoulder to shoulder, like someone who really cares, the quality of their communication grows to the extent that the patient regains a sense of joy, hope and faith, or even his health, no matter how serious his illness to be treated.

There is no doubt that humanizing this important relationship will result in a more positive therapeutic outcome. This being the case, the patient knows that he is not alone in the battle to regain his health or to improve its quality. When this is not attainable, at least he will be able to add some more productive days or years to his life. Then a sense of hope is established because the patient feels supported by the doctor, who is compassionate enough to hold hands with the client and to express reassurance during the painful moments of sick days.

There is nothing more uplifting than to feel secure by the sense of hope and encouragement delivered by someone who does not only know about life and death, but also is compassionate enough to give LOVE.

As mentioned previously in this book, during the physician-patient communication process there is a unique opportunity for the internal evolvement of both. In working together, it is not only the client who benefits, but the physician as well. This is what happens when the medical doctor has already grown enough to acknowledge that he is not that "All Powerful Physician," who knows the solution for all the types of medical problems. To reach the position in which he is able to be less defensive and guarded before his patient, the medical professional must be, first, seriously committed to learn about himself and to evolve. Therefore, it is healthy for a doctor to admit his limitations as a human being and to recognize himself as a person holding scientific knowledge about life, but who are not OMNIPOTENT and UNFAILING in his expertise. Following this premise, the physician will be aware that it is plausible that he might make mistakes. Accepting these facts is a worthy contribution to the process of DEMYSTIFYING the figure of the doctor in this society.

It is always worthwhile to remember that before becoming a doctor, the person is first a human being. Consequently, he is subjected to the same physical, emotional and spiritual laws as his patients. Holding a medical degree does not promote anyone to an elite of "super beings" above the entire human race. This means that physicians do not have the prerogative to act as "Medical Deities," expecting to be worshipped by society. It is not being said here that doctors should not be applauded or recognized by their merits when delivering good services to their clientele. On the contrary, it is the natural development in this symbiotic partnership. This is what ordinarily takes place when the physician is able to perceive his patient as a whole. Then, he will focus on the somatic and psychological features of a disease without overlooking important areas of the patient's life that affect the balance of his health.

The struggles of life do not exempt anyone. Each person faces different segments of the battle, with a variety of scenarios and different degrees of intensities in his attempt to accomplish the task of living. However, no one is left out of the "war." Some make it more or less easily and others get lost amidst the confusion of their days. Doctors, as a part of a sophisticated and competitive community, are challenged in a very hard way by the nature of their work.

To keep perspective and balance in all areas of their lives is almost impossible. Even so, physicians hardly admit that they also are susceptible to failing or getting sick.

"The Omnipotent Physician" has trouble in viewing himself as a regular human being. He does "his best" to conceal any shortcoming that can "tarnish" his reputation of being "superior." Some live an artificial life deprived of self-love and with a very poor self-image, despite their apparent presumptuous attitude. Their days are a permanent make believe, just to keep a facade of "being the ones who are above the standards." The patients under his care are the ones who suffer the most painful consequences of being treated by a professional who lives in silent despair.

As the closing thoughts of this book, it is paramount to emphasize the authors' deep desire to direct a strong appeal to the colleagues, aiming to encourage them to cultivate the noble quality of being humble.

Indeed, it is necessary to be unpretentious enough to accept that it is part of the human experience for everyone to have diseases. Even doctors!

The following step is to seek professional help. It is time to remove the old taboo that physicians cannot get sick, be emotionally unbalanced or present any type of disorder that negates their image of being "omnipotent, omniscient and omnipresent."

So, "DOCTOR, HEAL THYSELF, FIRST!"

Yes! Heal yourself, cultivating the powerful feeling of self-love! By developing this positive attitude, you will be at the beginning of a new path of self-discovery and self-empowering. You will find out that you are a more complete human being than you thought you were!

Through love, directed first to yourself and secondly to your patient, you will wake up in him the powerful healing process that potentially exists in every living being. Even if you do not accomplish the ultimate goal of curing your patient, in the medical sense, you are somehow contributing to heal him at the spiritual level. This happens when he learns how to experience LOVE, HARMONY and PEACE.

LOVE WALKS IN AND OPENS THE DOOR WHEN ALL ELSE FAILS!

By changing yourself into a "MESSENGER" of unconditional love, not only you and the patient under your care benefit, but also MANKIND. This happens because a person in a loving state of mind is at peace and in a virtuous position to touch those around him.

You will be a living part in the process of REHUMANIZING the sacred mission of the medical profession, now so distant from its altruistic goals!

* * *

> **LOVE IS THE ANSWER TO EVERY HUMAN NEED!**

Improve Your Practice With Better Communications
by Neil Baum, M.D.

> Dr. Neil Baum is a urologist in New Orleans, speaker on physician marketing and author of *Marketing Your Clinical Practice*. This article appeared in the *American Medical News*, May 24/31, 1993. Used by permission of author.

Patients keep you rich or make your poor depending on the service you provide. The most important ingredient to good service is communication.

We often think good communication is proportional to the time spent with patients. The truth is that effective communication can be accomplished in a short time if we focus on being good communicators and listeners.

In today's medical environment, health plans are squeezing access to physicians, the range of services covered and the time you spend with patients. That means you have more potential issues to deal with in less time.

At the same time, as markets become more competitive and patients more informed and demanding, patient satisfaction is growing in importance. Satisfied customers tell two to three potential patients about our services. Unfortunately, most physicians never hear from more than 90% of their unhappy patients, and dissatisfied patients tell 10 to 20 other people about what they didn't like. When we lose patient, it costs us as much as six times more to attract a new one than it did to attract the one we lost.

One factor that leads to patient attrition is poor communication, but few physicians take measures to ensure effective communication. Yet taking time to build and maintain patient relationships is a critical part of our jobs. When we don't communicate well, we miss valuable marketing opportunities. Now, more than ever, successful physicians are taking steps necessary to ensure patient satisfaction.

This month, with the help of Kittie Watson, Ph.D., a patient-physician communication specialist, I want to suggest four ways to improve patient communication. Dr. Watson is executive vice president of SPECTRA Communication Associates, former chair and associate professor in the Department of Communication at Tulane University, and co-author of such books as *Effective Listening: Key to Your Success and Relational Communication.*

Patient fears, nonverbal signals

Our patients come to us with medical problems. They look

to us for advice and solutions, but often feel insecure. They may have never had a medical problem before, feel embarrassed to discuss personal issues, question doctor-patient confidentiality or have body shyness. We often forget how it feels to be a patient.

Like many of us, patients don't like to admit that there is something wrong. They also don't like to admit their ignorance. Instead of asking for clarification, many patients, who are intimidated or afraid to ask questions, remain quiet. As physicians, we tend to over-estimated our patients' understanding of medical terminology and diagnoses.

We need to recognize nonverbal messages that may indicate discomfort, a lack of understanding or confusion. A patient who begins scratching his arm, pulling on an ear or touching his face while you're talking is probably feeling some anxiety.

When you notice such a behavior, think about what you can do to make the patient feel more comfortable. Consider asking a question, rephrasing what you said or asking for patient feedback. Keep in mind that similar nonverbal messages can have more than one meaning. A patient may have her arms crossed in front of her because she feels defensive, scared, cold or uncomfortable.

Check with each patient to make sure that you're interpreting a nonverbal signal correctly. When checking for understanding, avoid asking questions than can be answered with yes or no answers. Rather than asking, "Do you understand?" ask, "Which options are you willing to try?"

Build patient rapport

Get as much information as possible about a patient before seeing him or her for the first time. Getting office personnel to ask specific questions and create patient information files will save you time and build relationships more quickly. During your initial patient meeting, take specific notes. Be sure to include personal information such as marital status, number of children, hobbies and occupation.

Have your office staff organize your notes for you after each session. Review the patient's file before each appointment and use the information in your patient meetings. A quick review will remind you that some patients need to chat personally for a few minutes before giving medical information while others want to discuss their symptoms immediately. Learn to adapt your communication style to the individual needs of each patient.

While many physicians are very caring and concerned, they often don't get credit for it. Physicians show mixed messages when they don't demonstrate interest or involvement verbally and nonverbally. Be attentive and display concern through appropriate facial expressions such as smiles, raised eyebrows, and eye contact. To avoid making the wrong impression, pay more attention to the patient than your charts, diagnostic tests or next appointments. The first 15 seconds of a meeting are the most important for building relationships and making patients feel at ease. Be sure to shake hands and look each patient in the eye. Looking at patients more than at their files demonstrates your interest in them. Other ways to show interest and that you're listening include: leaning forward slightly, putting distracting objects out of reach, and responding to patient comments.

Make patients feel important

Treat each patient with respect. You can show respect by asking each patient how they prefer to be addressed. Don't assume all patients want to be called by their first or last names. Some patients, like physicians, have titles they prefer to use, such as colonel or doctor. Another way to show respect is to provide privacy for office conversations. Make sure patients can't overhear confidential conversations in waiting or examination rooms. Patients lose confidence in their physicians when they feel another patient's privacy has been violated.

Show patients that you value their time. Be sure to acknowledge delays and waiting times. Strive for promptness and show general courtesy when delays are inevitable. Listen to what the patient has to say. Don't discount their feelings and concerns. Even if a concern isn't justified, take time to hear the message, give specific feedback and make appropriate responses. Treating each patient with respect helps him or her maintain a sense of dignity in uncomfortable situations.

Train your staff

In your absence, office personnel provide first impressions of you and your services. While employees realize the importance of making good impressions during employment interviews, many fail to maintain polished images once they're hired. Employees who are careless about business etiquette, office neatness, personal appearance and language create negative first impressions that may cost you a client. Since office staffs are precursors to physicians, it is important for them to display the image you want.

Make sure your staff is trained in how you want them to come across. Coach receptionists in how to greet patients on the phone and in person. Instead of saying, "Dr. Smith's office," teach them to say, "Good morning, Dr. Smith's office. This is Ruby. How may I help you?"

Since most communication habits were established and reinforced long before you became a physician, changing and creating new habits isn't easy. We have to make special efforts to be sure that we have successfully communicated with our patients. There's no better way to make patients feel satisfied with their health care providers than to place a high priority on effective patient communication.

HOMESCHOOLING BOOKS by BLUE BIRD PUBLISHING
Order Form on Back Page

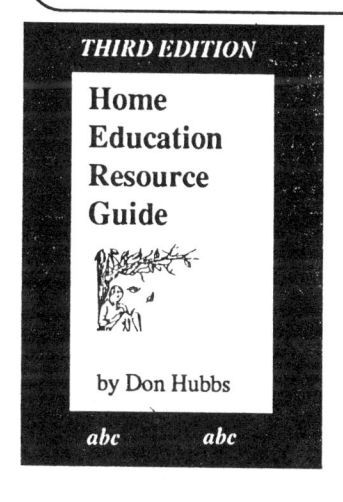

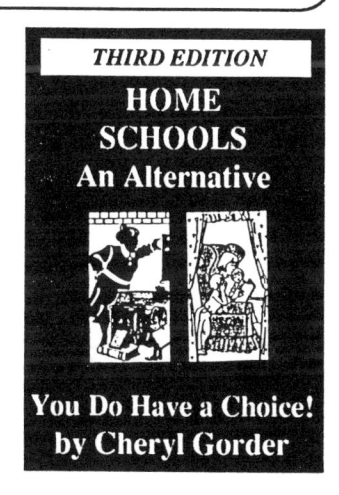

THIRD EDITION
Home Education Resource Guide
by Don Hubbs
abc   abc

THIRD EDITION
HOME SCHOOLS
An Alternative
You Do Have a Choice!
by Cheryl Gorder

LIBRARY JOURNAL— Feb. 1, 1995

"If you can afford only one resource directory, this is the one to buy."—about Home Education Resource Guide. ISBN 0-933025-25-4 $11.95.

"Includes an excellent summary of the reasons parents cite for their dissatisfaction with public schools and decision to homeschool."—about Home Schools: An Alternative. ISBN 0-933025-18-1 $11.95.

BOTH TITLES ARE HOMESCHOOLING BESTSELLERS AND IN THIRD EDITION.

Available from Baker & Taylor

MORE FAMILY ISSUES BOOKS by BLUE BIRD PUBLISHING

THE O.J. SYNDROME
CONFESSIONS OF AN ABUSER
by Rich Bean and Karen Crane

Every 12 seconds a woman is battered. 75% of women killed by the man they love are killed while trying to leave. It is estimated that as many as 4,000 women die each year at the hands of their domestic partners.
IT'S TIME TO DO SOMETHING ABOUT THE O.J. SYNDROME!
    Rich Bean and his daughter, Karen Crane, have written a touching, yet true, story about Rich Bean's tragic years as an abuser and his recovery. It's a story that may spare someone from such horrors.
ISBN 0-933025-39-4 $11.95

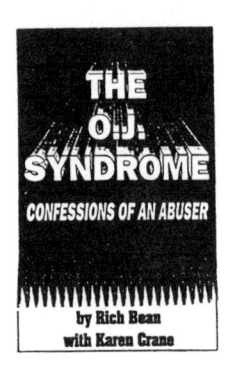

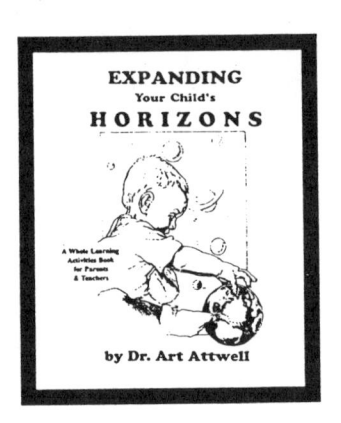

Expanding Your Child's HORIZONS
A Whole Learning Activities Book for Parents & Teachers
by Dr. Art Attwell

    Parents and teachers need to develop children who can become all they can be—children whose inquiring minds are appreciated and encouraged, whose creative ideas are not stifled. That's the purpose of whole learning.
    This book contains over a hundred activities that can be easily used in the home or classroom with simple materials. The activities are designed to help children develop self-esteem, creativity, an inner focus, intuition, joy and pleasure in learning, and problem-solving skills.
ISBN 0-933025-28-9 $12.95

> **MORE HOMESCHOOLING BOOKS by BLUE BIRD PUBLISHING**
> Order Form on Back Page

ROAD SCHOOL
by the Marousis Family

Many people dream, but few people pursue those dreams. Many hope for a better education for their children, but few do anything about it. This is the story of one family who did both.

In September of 1993, the Jim and Janet Marousis left Craig, Alaska, with $12,000, their pickup truck, and their daughters, Kaitlin, 10, and Jordin, 8. They began to "Road School" their daughters—and each other. This is the account of their adventures—of learning, changing, adapting, pleasures and disappointments.
ISBN 0-933025-36-X $14.95

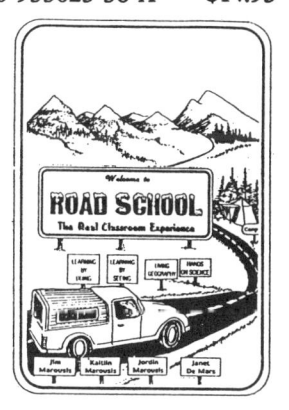

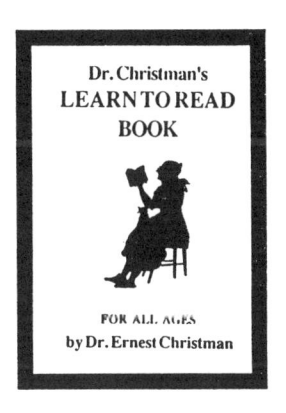

Dr. Christman's Learn to Read Book

With just this one book, a person can teach anyone to read! It's true because people tell us about it every day! Here are some of the unsolicited comments we have heard at the office:

"I absolutely love this book!"—Carol Sanford, literacy volunteer at Aspen Prison.

"I teach as a volunteer for the literacy program. This book works very well. I am teaching a 60-year-old man who has never read in his life."—Mary Saxon.

"Best book for learning English ever!"—Tom Evans, asking to translate this book for use by Koreans.
ISBN 0-933025-17-3 $15.95

ORDER FORM

To order more books from Blue Bird Publishing, use this handy order form. To receive a free catalog of all of the current titles (parenting, homeschooling, educational, relationships, and more), please send business size SASE to address below.

_____	*Improving the Doctor-Patient Relationship*	$11.95
_____	*Divorced Dad's Handbook*	$12.95
_____	*Home Schools: An Alternative (3rd Ed)*	$11.95
_____	*Home Education Resource Guide (3rd Ed)*	$11.95
_____	*Road School*	$14.95
_____	*The O.J. Syndrome: Confessions of an Abuser*	$11.95
_____	*Dragon-Slaying for Couples*	$14.95
_____	*Parent's Solution to a Problem Child*	$11.95
_____	*Dr. Christman's Learn-to-Read Book*	$15.95
_____	*Survival Guide to Step-Parenting*	$11.95
_____	*Preschool Learning Activities*	$15.95

Shipping charges: $2.50 for first book.
Add 50¢ for each additional book.
Total charges for books:_____
Total shipping charges:_____
TOTAL ENCLOSED:_____

NAME:_____
ADDRESS:_____
CITY, STATE, ZIP:_____
Telephone #: _____
For Credit Card Order:
   Card #:_____
   Expiration Date:_____

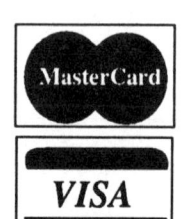

Send mail order to:
BLUE BIRD PUBLISHING
1739 East Broadway #306
Tempe AZ 85282
(602) 968-4088   (602) 831-6063